Your First
JIRD

CONTENTS

Photographs by:
**Paul Davis,
Melissa V Page,
Frank Naylor,
Karin van Veen (Persian Jirds)**

Front cover painting by:
D A Lish

INTRODUCTION

The purpose of this book is to give a helping hand to new owners of pet jirds. So little is known about jirds that no book devoted solely to the species has ever been published before. Where possible I have drawn on what scientific facts are available, but the vast majority of information is taken from my many years' experience of keeping rodents, jirds in particular.

For the purpose of this book, 'jird' refers to the species commonly available in the United Kingdom – the Shaw's Jird (Meriones shawi shawi). The Shaw's Jird looks like a giant gerbil and is a close relative of the so-called Mongolian Gerbil – which in fact is not a gerbil at all but a jird (Meriones unguiculatus or Clawed Jird)!

Another species of jird, already available to breeders in Continental Europe and expected soon to arrive in the fancy in the United Kingdom, is the Persian Jird (Meriones persicus).

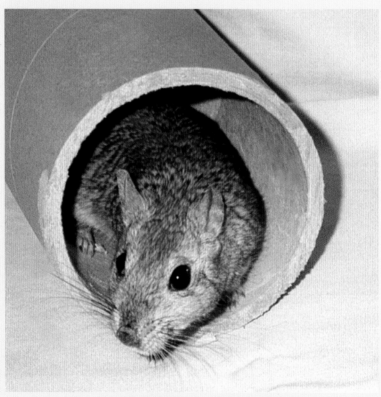

**In the wild, jirds are burrowing creatures,
and this Shaw's Jird is enjoying playing in a cardboard tube.**

Shaw's Jird originates from the warm, arid areas of North Africa: Morocco, Algeria, Libya, Egypt and Tunisia. It has about the same size of body as a rat and makes its burrow underground in hard clay, usually beneath shrubs. The burrow can be up to a metre (3ft) deep and always has numerous entrances, affording the jird a choice of escape routes should some predator such as a snake find its way into the burrow. Shaw's Jirds come in only one colour, classed as agouti, although this varies from yellowish to brownish tones in individuals. It gradually shades to a lighter, creamy colour on the belly.

The female jird is extremely dominant and territorial and will only accept a male into her burrow when she is on heat. Males, although generally more placid, will fight each other viciously when competing for females. Such fights often result in less dominant males being injured, or even killed in extreme cases.

Once mated, the female carries her young for a period of 21 days before giving birth in the relative safety of the burrow. For the next three weeks, she feeds her young and tends to their every need, leaving them only for short spells to forage. By the fourth week, the youngsters venture out of the burrow to explore the outside world. Shortly after this, the mother loses interest in her young and often refuses to let them back into the burrow, thus forcing them to make their own way in the world.

The Persian Jird is found in an area extending from Eastern Turkey to Pakistan. It is slightly larger than Shaw's Jird and prefers a rocky environment, building its nest between boulders. When it has to burrow, it does not go deeper than a metre. The gestation period of 28 days is longer than that of the Shaw's Jird. Its colour is warmer, with chestnut tones, and there is a definite border between the dark, shiny top colour and the white belly.

Distinguishing between the sexes is very easy. One indication is that the male tends to be heavier in build than the female and, as he gets older, to develop bulges on his cheeks. However, the real deciding factor is the large scrotal sack situated at the base of the male's tail.

In the wild the jird's diet consists of seeds, grains and green leaves. Jirds will also eat fruit, berries and, sometimes, insects.

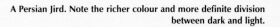

A Persian Jird. Note the richer colour and more definite division between dark and light.

HOUSING

When you first buy your jird you will probably have a recently-weaned infant little more than the size of a gerbil. Remember when purchasing a home for your jird that this little animal will soon reach the size of a pet rat.

The average body length of an adult jird is 140–145mm (about 5^1/$_2$in) with the tail also reaching approximately 140mm. It would be false economy to buy a tank or cage that would soon be outgrown. The Persian Jird is slightly larger, at 145–168mm (5^1/$_2$–6^1/$_2$in) with a tail of up to 188mm (7^1/$_2$in)

Siting

The siting of the tank or cage is very important. It is vital to place it where there is no risk of it overheating. The dangers to watch out for are:
- heat from direct sources such as radiators and fires
- heat from indirect sources such as sunlight through a window

It is equally important that jirds should not be subjected to cold and draughts. I would advise jird owners in the United Kingdom and other countries where the weather is changeable not to keep jirds outside in hutches.

Aquariums (tanks)

A tank is an ideal home for your jird. Size and cost vary greatly but it is far better to buy the largest tank you can afford. The minimum size for a pair of jirds is 90cm x 37.5cm x 37.5cm (36in x 15in x 15in), larger if possible.

A tank gives you a great deal of scope. You can furnish the interior with tubes, tunnels, ceramic containers and so on, and then cover the base with a deep layer of wood shavings. Any tank will require a tight-fitting cover. Wire mesh sheets with a grid size of 12mm x 12mm are ideal if you want to make your own. If not, you can purchase a ready-made lid (the type normally used for vivariums) from a pet shop. This type of lid will keep out intruders while allowing adequate ventilation.

The main advantage of using a glass tank is that it limits mess. Jirds love to have a 'How far can we throw our wood shavings?' competition every night.

Another advantage is that tanks with close-fitting lids are difficult to escape from, and jirds are natural escape artists. They are immensely strong for their size and more intelligent than most of the other species of rodent I have kept over the years.

Cages

You can also house your jirds in cages. Pet shops stock cages in a variety of shapes and sizes. As with most things, you get what you pay for, and it is certainly worth purchasing the largest, best quality cage you can afford.

The smallest cage I would recommend for a pair of jirds is the modern chinchilla cage, which measures approximately 63cm x 40cm x 68cm. This type of cage has a deep plastic tray, easily detached for cleaning. The upper part of the cage is made of steel bars and the cage is available in a range of finishes,

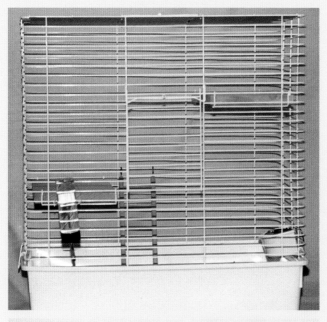

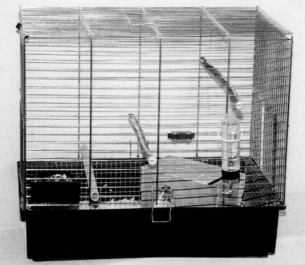

A chinchilla cage (top) makes an ideal home for a jird,
as does a converted cockatiel cage (below).

usually plastic-coated or chrome-plated. Always check the finish of the bars for rough edges or uneven coating, and bear in mind that cheaper quality chrome plating will soon rust. A jird will certainly test the quality of any cage you buy by gnawing the bars constantly. If the chrome deteriorates to such an extent that rust starts to form, cleaning the bars will be difficult and dirt and bacteria will collect on the rough surface of the steel bars. Should your jird continue to gnaw on these bars, there is a risk that an open sore or wound will develop on its snout, often leading to an infection.

Juna tanks

Another type of housing you might like to try is a Juna tank. I have used these and found them to be excellent. They are available in a range of sizes and each consists of a thick plastic base and a clear cover made from heavy-duty perspex. The cover has a removable coated metal grill, to allow the jird to breathe.

This accommodation is ideal for young jirds as there is little chance of them hurting themselves in it. I also find that this type of housing allows you more freedom in deciding where to place the cage since, because of its design, there is very little mess. You can totally strip the cage for easy cleaning which is very important. I have also found this type of cage to be virtually escape proof – definitely a bonus!

Cleaning

The tank or cage – together with nest box, food bowls, bottle and everything else – should be cleaned out at least once a week, twice in hot, humid weather. I half-fill a bucket reserved solely for the jirds with warm water to which I have added a capful of Dettol (to halt the build-up of bacteria) and a dash of washing-up liquid. Using a damp cloth, I wipe the inside of the tank or cage until it is really clean and then dry it with a separate cloth. I leave it to 'air' for 5–10 minutes and then put in fresh woodshavings and clean nesting material, followed by fresh food and water. Once everything is ready, I

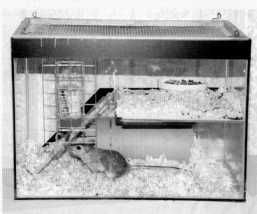

An aquarium set-up.
Tanks are particularly good at containing the mess when jirds decide to throw sawdust around.

put the jirds back in. It is worth noting that newly-weaned young may well need their home to be cleaned out more often, as they tend to be messy.

If the jird's water bottle is subjected to sunlight, algae will soon form on the inner surface. This can be removed easily with a bottle brush.

Warning – Wheels Avoid the use of wheels in both tanks and cages. More often than not they cause serious injuries to the tail and feet, either of which can so easily become trapped.

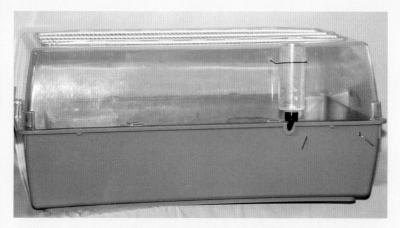

A Juna tank: ideal for keeping young jirds.

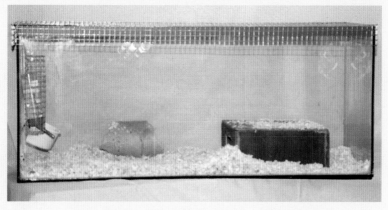

Another aquarium set-up. Note the mesh lid – vital for security.

SUBSTRATE AND BEDDING

Various materials are available as floor coverings and bedding for your jirds, and I shall discuss the most usual ones below:

Floor covering (substrate)

The choice of materials to cover the base of your tank or cage is, in my opinion, limited to three alternatives: sawdust, peat and woodshavings. I shall try to list the advantages and disadvantages of each.

Sawdust

Sawdust is cheap and readily available. It can be obtained in a pre-packed form from pet shops or bought loose from sawmills and timber-yards.

I feel that, because of its fine consistency, sawdust has many disadvantages. Admittedly, it readily and easily soaks up moisture and urine, but it just as readily coagulates, firstly into large clumps and then into a solid mass. Very soon the absorption of liquid ceases and the sawdust is incapable of carrying out the task for which it is intended.

If you decide to use sawdust to cover the base of your tank or cage, bear in mind that you will have to ensure the well-being of your pet by cleaning out the cage regularly and painstakingly.

Other problems with sawdust from a jird's point of view – bearing in mind that a jird is very clean, and fastidious in its toilet habits – are:

Odour: Urine, as we all know, gives off an offensive smell. Within the confines of a cage or tank, this smell soon intensifies as the sawdust becomes more and more laden with moisture. As the medium compacts, air cannot pass freely between the fine particles to dissipate the smell, so the atmosphere becomes very unpleasant for the jirds.

Burying the drinking bottle's outlet: Jirds love to dig. In a matter of minutes, what was a nice, level layer of sawdust is a large mound up one side of the cage or tank. If the drinking bottle is in the line of fire and the bottle's outlet is covered in sawdust, in a very short space of time the bottle is drained. This means that not only does your pet not have a drink until you refill the bottle but the water that was in the bottle soaks into the cage or tank bottom. This soon leads to the formation of mildew, which in turn gives off a horrible, stale, musty smell. If this happens, the tank or cage must be emptied, cleaned thoroughly and then disinfected to kill off any bacteria that may have built up.

Irritation: Sawdust in its dry state gives off a very fine dust. The particles can easily irritate the eyes, nose or skin of your jird.

Peat

I have never used peat as a tank or cage floor covering but I know several people who have. Some of these claim it to be a wonderful substance; others claim it is of no use at all. If peat is your choice, I would advise you to mix it with another substance to give it some structure, and I think woodshavings are the ideal material for this purpose. It is only practical to use peat in a glass tank, and it will be necessary to check regularly that the peat does not become water-logged. This can happen very rapidly in a glass tank and even short exposure to this problem can result in serious health risks for your pet, notably skin problems and foot rot, neither of which is pleasant and both of which urgently require veterinary treatment.

Woodshavings

It may seem from this section that I am biased towards woodshavings – and I am. Over many years of keeping various species of rodent, including jirds, rats, gerbils and chinchillas, I have found this medium far better than all others.

To ensure the quality of the woodshavings, always buy them from a reputable source, such as from your pet supplier. Savings come in handy-sized packs suitable for owners of one small pet right up to giant-sized bales for horse-owners. These are often bought by breeders like myself, as they represent good value for money.

Warning: always check through your woodshavings for large splinters of wood. If these are not removed from your pet's cage, wounds and eye damage can easily occur.

I have found woodshavings to be absorbent and heat retentive. Generally they do not compact and they are easy to dispose of. I have also found that they tend to combat the problem of odour, and I believe this is because the air can pass freely through the large particles.

Bedding

Shredded paper is ideal bedding for newborn babies and infants.

You can also buy bedding made from special fibres, with the appearance and texture of cotton wool. This is fine for use with adult jirds but I would not recommend it for newborn babies – it tends to stick to their skin.

These and many other kinds can be purchased from most pet shops. At the end of the day, the choice of bedding is down to you and, to some extent, to your jird.

You can also let your pet make its own bedding by providing a good supply of toilet tissue, kitchen roll, soft tissues, and so on. This will not only give your jird a nice soft bed but also provide hours of entertainment as it shreds, rips and shapes it to its heart's content.

FURNISHING

Your jird is an intelligent animal that needs stimulation. A bare, unfurnished home would soon cause your pet to become bored and unhappy.

I would advise people to avoid buying expensive objects such as push-together tubing, because jirds, like any other rodents, love to chew. Animals do not understand the value of money; irrespective of whether an item costs 10p or £10, the jird just views it as something to chew on!

You can create an interesting home for your jird by giving it different objects to play with. Simple things like the insides of toilet rolls will be gnawed and used as toys and are easily and cheaply replaced. Old tissue boxes with a few tissues left in them can also be used. You could add any soft paper such as kitchen roll. Any of these items will fascinate your jird, who will shred and chew them and add them to his or her bedding. Avoid thin plastic toys because, as your jird gnaws them, small pieces may be swallowed, with possibly fatal consequences. The same applies to soft rubber toys. You can also buy an assortment of toys from most pet shops, but remember that any toys should be large enough for a fully grown jird either to turn around in or pass through.

You can furnish your jird's tank quite cheaply if you shop around. Simple objects such as thick cardboard tubing cut into small lengths are ideal for your jird to gnaw on. Certain fish tank ornaments also can be used. One I have tried is ceramic glazed piping with a central opening, approximately 20cm (8in) in length and 10cm (4in) in diameter. Jirds have a great time running in and out of it. Other items worth trying are clay plant pots, but only new ones should be used. Ceramic glazed 'boots' are good, too. They have a top opening and often an open toe end, and my jirds love them.

Most of the items mentioned can be found around the house or purchased from pet shops and garden centres.

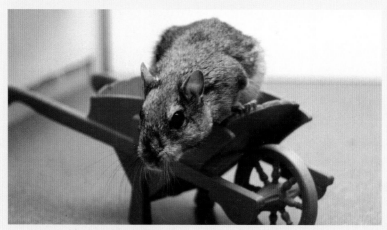

A Shaw's Jird exploring an ornamental wheel barrow.

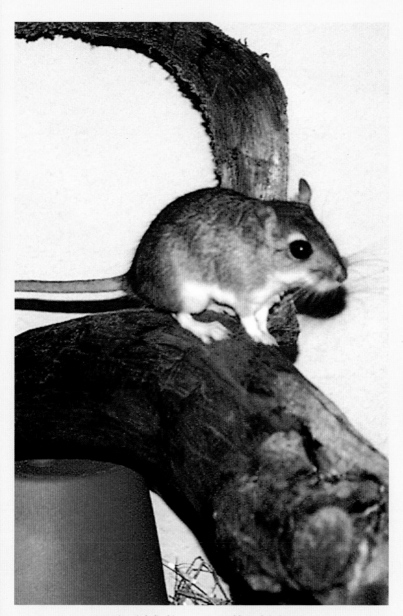

A Persian Jird climbing on a natural branch in its cage.

HANDLING

A jird that is handled regularly soon becomes tame. Jirds recognise you and respond to the sound of your voice once they have become accustomed to you.

Before handling your jird, make sure it has seen you. Never put your hand straight in to pick it up. Naturally, if your jird is startled, it will become defensive. I always talk to my jirds before I handle them so that they know I am there.

When handling a jird, always make sure that you use the base of the tail only to restrain them, not as a 'handle', and support the rest of the body with your other hand. Never lift a jird out of the cage or tank solely by its tail, especially by the middle or end of the tail. If you do this, the skin can easily become detached, leaving just bone and a great deal of blood. If this happens, veterinary help must be sought immediately.

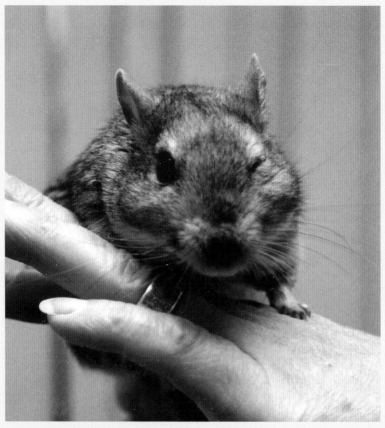

If you handle your jird regularly, it will soon become tame.

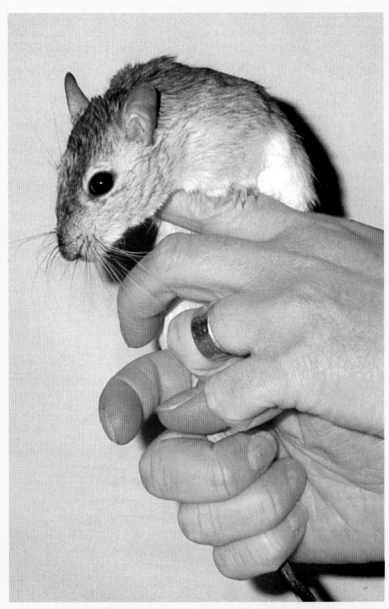

You can restrain your jird by holding the base of the tail, but never pick a jird up by the tail.

FEEDING

Any rodent needs a well-balanced diet, and jirds are no exception. You will find out which foods to offer by trial and error. Your jird will definitely let you know which are its favourites!

Mixes

You must provide a food mixture that gives your jird lots of energy and keeps it in tip-top condition. You can obtain a good variety of gerbil and hamster mixes that will meet most of your pet's dietary needs. The mix contains a vast assortment of dried food items such as oats, wheat, peanuts, flaked peas, barley, and sunflower seeds.

Additions to the mix

You can add other foods to your hamster and gerbil mix. Locust nuts and a mix of small biscuits are much appreciated by jirds. Sunflower seeds are a favourite; they will eat one after another. Yes, sunflower seeds are fattening, but I have never experienced a jird with a weight problem. They only eat the amount they need.

I have found that jirds like small amounts of bread, plain crackers, digestive biscuits and even breadsticks. Jirds also love raisins.

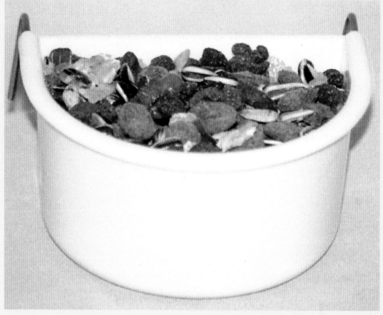

Hamster mix in a bowl that will hang on the side of the cage.

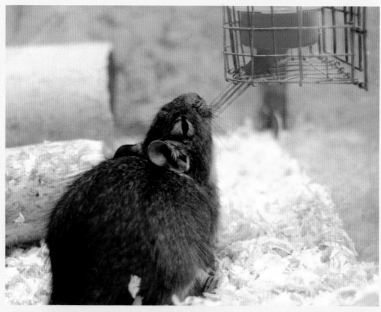

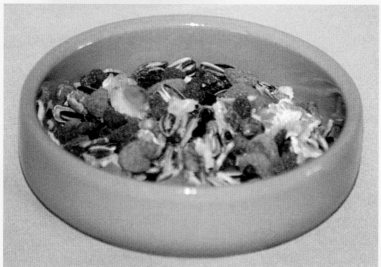

(Above) a jird enjoying a drink from the water bottle, and
(below) a heavy ceramic dish containing hamster mix.

Fresh fruits and vegetables

I supplement my jirds' diet with a variety of fresh fruits at least twice a week for additional vitamins and minerals. In captivity, your jird cannot forage for fruit and berries so it is up to you to supply them for your pet. Before offering your pet any fruit or vegetables, make sure the produce has been washed thoroughly. This a precaution because almost all fruit and vegetables are sprayed with insecticides.

I must strongly advise against the use of unidentified berries you find in the garden or hedgerow. Many kinds of berry are highly poisonous and must not be given. However, you can give vegetables along with fruit as dietary supplements.

Safe fruits to offer are small amounts of apple, grapes, banana, pears, peaches, dried apricot, coconut (fresh, not desiccated), dried cherries, raisins and kiwi fruit (sliced). Never give citrus fruits as these easily cause stomach upsets. The vegetables I suggest are peas in the pod, lettuce, carrots, parsnips and watercress.

When to feed

You will probably have read in other books about rodents that you should feed them only at certain times of the day when the animals are active. Jirds differ from most other rodents as they are not strictly nocturnal – they are busy throughout the day as well as night. You would have a very upset jird if its food dish was not available at all times.

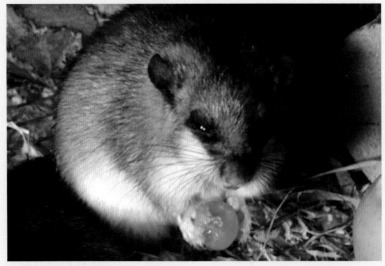

A jird enjoying a grape. Jirds like their food to be available at all times.

BREEDING

As you become more used to jirds, you may decide to breed your own stock.

Selecting your breeding stock

At present, jirds are a relatively unknown species. This means that they are expensive to buy and difficult to obtain. However, if the popularity of this rodent is to increase, breeders must use only the best quality animals.

As a breeder of jirds I know just how difficult it is to find stockists who even know what jirds are, let alone sell them. I would advise any potential buyer to look very carefully at the jirds' surroundings in the pet shop:

- Is the area clean and tidy?
- Is there a good supply of food and water?

If these are satisfactory then look at the general health of the jird. Don't be afraid to pick up the animal. Look closely at the following points:

- Is its coat smooth and glossy with no lumps or bumps?
- Are the eyes bright and shiny?
- Are the nose and mouth clear of any discharge?
- Are the anus and genital area clean and dry?
- Are there any deformities (for instance, kinks in the tail)?
- Are all the limbs present?
- Does the animal seem alert and active?

A word of advice: do not buy two jirds from the same supplier as a breeding pair because, more often than not, you will have purchased a brother and sister. You need to start with unrelated stock. I have seen first hand what another breeder achieved from inbreeding: a male from the litter was born with a club foot and a female with one eye. She was rescued by me as no one else wanted her. If there are already faults in a line, breeding from close relatives makes it much more likely that they will surface in the litter.

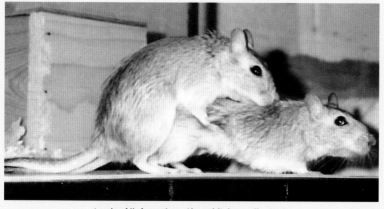

A pair of jirds mating – if you blink, you'll miss it!

Do-it-yourself nest box

Before you start the process of breeding jirds, you will need to prepare a nest box to put in their cage. The nest box should be of a generous size. It is no use providing your pets with a home that they will rapidly outgrow.

The following plans are copied from the design I use for my own jirds.

Size

I have found that the ideal size for a nest box (see diagram A) is:
    250mm wide x 225mm deep x 100mm high, or 10in x 9in x 4in.

Material

Ideally, the box should be made from wood and I have found 13mm plywood to be the best choice. I have to warn you to be prepared to replace the nest box regularly. It is quite amazing how quickly a jird can destroy even thick plywood with their teeth.

Cutting list

    2 pieces 250mm x   225mm (base and lid)
    2 pieces 250mm x   100mm (front and back)
    2 pieces 225mm x   100mm (sides)
    2 pieces 19mm   x   19mm softwood (lid guides)

Construction

Take one of the 250mm x 100mm pieces of plywood and cut a doorway in it as shown in diagram B. Fit this piece and the other piece which measures the same to the base by means of small nails.

Take the two pieces that measure 200mm x 100mm and fit them to the base. You should now have the main part of your nest box.

Now fit the two pieces of 19mm x 19mm softwood to the last piece of plywood, which measures 250mm x 225mm, as shown in diagram C.

A quick rub down with sandpaper to remove any splinters or rough edges, and your new nest box is ready.

The female's cycle

A female jird is capable of mating all the year round. There is no technical reference available on the subject but, from my own observations, I would estimate it to be a four-week cycle. The signs that she is ready to mate are as follows:
- She will scent mark much more than usual to let passing males know that she is ready to mate.
- She will stamp her feet repeatedly on any hard surface she can find.

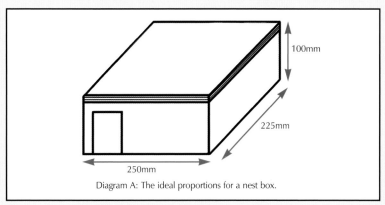

Diagram A: The ideal proportions for a nest box.

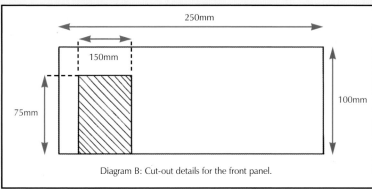

Diagram B: Cut-out details for the front panel.

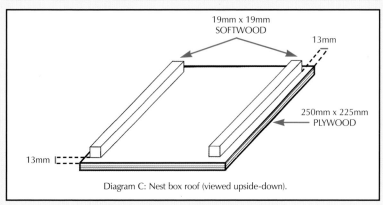

Diagram C: Nest box roof (viewed upside-down).

Do-it-yourself nest box.

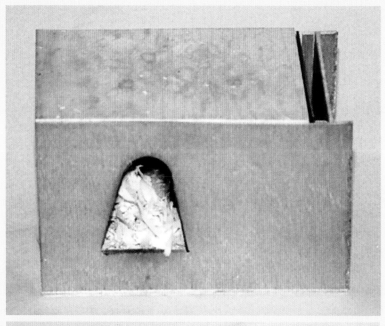

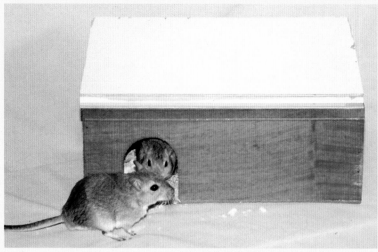

(Above) a converted, shop-bought nest box (entrance altered) and
(below) a home-made box, with occupants.

She will carry on with this behaviour for several days until either she finds a mate or the urge to mate subsides. If you have two females living together and one of them comes on heat, she will very probably try to mate her companion, assuming the position usually adopted by the male. This is normal behaviour – nothing to worry about.

Pairing off

Unlike most other rodents, jirds are pedantic in their choice of partners. They will not always readily accept a mate chosen for them.

When you first introduce male to female, it should be on neutral ground – not in a confined space such as the tank or cage belonging to one of them. In the room where I keep my jirds, I have a large, U-shaped worktop. When I introduce prospective partners, normally I put the male one end and the female the other, so that they can meet when they are ready. They begin by sniffing the area, and then they sniff each other. Usually, what follows can be best described as 'trial by ordeal'. To the inexperienced observer their behaviour looks particularly aggressive, with both animals rearing up to their full height on their rear legs and engaging in what bears a close resemblance to a boxing match.

This performance is a test of strength. If the male is defeated by the female, she will not consider him a suitable partner and they will go on sparring until they are separated from each other. If the match goes the other way and the male overpowers the female, this is a good sign that you have a potential breeding pair. When things seem settled, introduce them to their new home together.

I would suggest you still keep a close eye on them. At first there will still be what looks like chaos, and this can go on for several hours while they are getting to know each other.

If the jirds decide that they are going to accept each other the next stage usually is grooming. You will see the animals take it in turn to lick and clean each other. If the female is satisfied that the male is suitable, mating will occur.

Mating

Blink and you will have missed your jirds mating – it is literally that quick! In the wild, it has been recorded that a pair will mate approximately 224 times in a space of two hours. In captivity, the number of matings will be many fewer, as the risk of becoming lunch for some other creature is removed. Even so, the pair will still copulate throughout the day and night, and this can, and often does, go on for days.

The jirds have now formed a bond which, on the female's part, is monogamous. Not so the male – he will chance his luck with any other female he may happen across.

Two females will live quite happily with one male jird, provided that they are of a similar, young age when they are introduced, but never try this the opposite way round, putting two males with one female. Male jirds are extremely territorial, especially when there are females around, and keeping two within the close confines of a tank or cage will result in serious injury or possibly the death of the weaker animal.

One problem with a male jird is that he can be too amorous for his own good. If he persists in his attempts at mounting the female when she is no longer interested, more often than not she will turn on him very aggressively, and then he can end up with nasty injuries.

Pregnancy

The female jird reaches sexual maturity at about 12 weeks, but the male jird can reproduce at about five weeks. The gestation period is 21 days from conception.

Although a female jird will allow a male to mount her from a few weeks old, it is highly unlikely that she will conceive much before she is 12 weeks old. However, this is only a guideline: there are exceptions to any rule.

Before you decide to breed your jirds, the female must be in the very best of health. You can prepare a female by providing the diet necessary to build up her body reserves, as the processes of pregnancy, giving birth and rearing offspring are physically demanding.

The pair should take a good amount of exercise. This is only possible if you have provided them with a large enough tank or cage. The female's diet can be adjusted accordingly. Her food should contain a high protein content. This could be in the form of evaporated milk with small amounts of bread added. Do not worry if the male decides to help himself to whatever is on offer. Provided that the female gets her share, it really does not matter. Carry on with this method of feeding until she has finished nursing her young and then return them slowly to their normal diet.

Before returning your female to her normal diet, make sure she has not mated again since the birth of her last litter. If you are not sure, keep her on a well balanced diet. You can still give her small amounts of fruit and vegetables.

The female shows very little evidence of being pregnant. Towards the end of her pregnancy you may notice a slight swelling of her stomach area. Occasionally, you may see a swelling of her nipples in preparation for producing milk for her young.

Birth

The female usually gives birth during late evening or in the early hours of the morning. She does not normally require any assistance in giving birth – the whole process is over in a very short space of time.

Care of the litter

The average litter numbers two to four infants. Once the mother has given birth, it is vital that the nest box is not disturbed or cleaned. If it becomes necessary to move the babies for any reason, you must wear latex gloves so that your scent does not pass onto the infants. Failure to do this can result in the mother abandoning the babies, who will then die very quickly through lack of nourishment. I do not disturb the nest box or the rest of the cage or tank until the young are safely past 21 days old.

Newborn jirds are blind, helpless, naked and deaf. Hair growth is very rapid and within a week they have a full coat. By 10 days the ears have formed and by 14 days the eyes will have opened. At this point, the babies are more than capable of leaving the nest and they will start to explore their surroundings. The mother is still extremely protective of her youngsters and will often be seen running around after them. She will pick up each baby in turn and carry it back to the nest box in her mouth. This seems an endless process for the mother. When the young are three weeks old, the mother becomes far more relaxed about looking after them, but she will still return them to the safety of the nest box if she feels there is a threat of danger.

Weaning

Baby jirds are weaned by the time they reach four weeks of age. The offspring tend to follow their mother's example, quickly learning how to use a drinking bottle and choose the tastiest morsels from the food dish.

Independence

It is advisable to separate the young into different sexes and house them away from the mother by the time they reach five weeks of age. This will minimise the risk of one of the male babies trying to mate with his own mother, and a juvenile male will repeatedly try to mate his sisters, although they are far too young to become pregnant.

Unwanted pregnancies

Male jirds actually serve very little purpose apart from mating to continue the species. The male does not get involved in the building of the nest and gives little or no help to the female in rearing the young. In fact, his presence is more of a hindrance to the female after she has given birth because of his repeated attempts at mating with her again. My method of preventing this problem from arising is to remove him altogether from the 'married quarters' before the birth, placing him in separate accommodation. A female jird can become pregnant again within seven days of giving birth to her litter; in fact she is very fertile during this seven days.

Allowing a female to have one litter after another not only places a great strain on her but also ultimately results in a loss of quality in the offspring. I do not allow my females to breed again for at least 10–12 weeks after they have given birth.

It is worth mentioning that the female's character sometimes undergoes a temporary change after the birth of her offspring. I believe that this is due to the increased hormonal activity in her body, which will return to normal over a period of 5–6 weeks. During this period she can sometimes 'nip' for no apparent reason.

Housing the youngsters

When the youngsters are weaned they should be put into separate accommodation. I separate the males from the females at 5–6 weeks, and then separate the males into pairs at about 8 weeks to minimise bullying of the weaker jirds. However, I would not advise placing a jird in a cage or tank by itself. Jirds are very social animals and need the company of their own kind.

The choice of 'room-mates' is always problematic, and it is definitely easier to introduce young jirds to each other. Individual temperaments vary considerably. As I have already said, two young females can usually be settled quite happily with a male of the same age, but introducing older males and females is less likely to be successful. Two adult males will sometimes live happily together if they are the same size and their temperaments are similar, although there will always be some tussles. They should always be introduced gradually, not just put in together and left to 'get on with it'. It should soon be clear whether they are going to get on with each other. Those introduced at 5–6 weeks old will very often live happily ever after.

Once you have separated the youngsters from their mother, it is important to watch them carefully for the next few days, just in case they are not yet fully independent. It is essential that the youngsters are fully weaned before being separated from their mother because there is no guarantee that she will accept them back again.

Keeping breeding records

I would advise anyone thinking of breeding jirds to keep detailed records. It is so easy to lose track, especially if you are breeding in large numbers. You can use a book, a breeding card system or a computer. Whichever method you decide to use, it will be invaluable for future reference.

If you are using a card system for breeding records, have a card for each mating and write on it the names of the pair, their ages, what kind of temperament each has, the number of offspring produced, how the mother cared for her young and whether all the youngsters were healthy. You should also include details on how the youngsters progressed: how old they were when they opened their eyes and became fully weaned and if they had any problems.

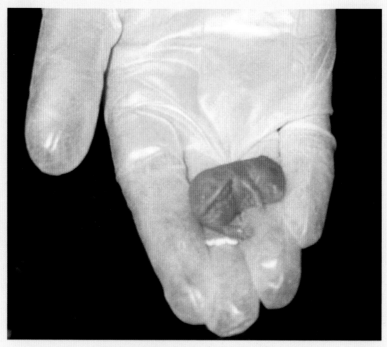

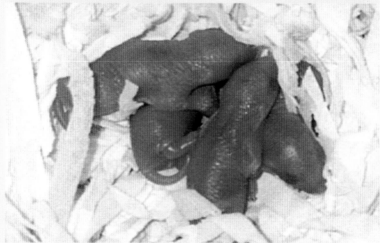

If possible, avoid disturbing or cleaning the nest box once the babies are born. If you have to move the babies for any reason, wear latex gloves so that the infants do not smell of you.

BEHAVIOUR

The jird has several specific habits that are interesting to observe. They are part of its daily life and you should look at what your pet is doing so that you can understand it better. None of the many different species of rodents I have kept over the years has proved more interesting to keep than the jird. I have found that the more time and effort you spend with your jird, the greater are the benefits.

I have been asked on numerous occasions, 'Do jirds make good pets?' The answer is, 'Yes, they make wonderful pets and are ideal for adults and children alike.'

Another question I have frequently been asked is whether a jird can be kept with other rodents. The answer is, 'No, they can only be kept with their own kind.'

Periods of activity

Jirds have good eyesight, a keen sense of smell and acute hearing. Unlike some rodents, they are not truly nocturnal and have periods of activity throughout the day and night. In an average litter there is always one who is far more adventurous and outgoing than all the others. This is the one that the mother will return to the nest box time and time again. On the other hand, there is always the timid one who needs that extra reassurance.

In the nest

A young jird starts showing individual behaviour from an early age, often as young as three weeks. Some of these patterns of behaviour are inborn, some are learnt from parents. Before the youngster even ventures out of the nest box, you will often hear the sounds of scratching and digging and, if you lift the lid of the nest box very gently, you may be lucky enough to see an infant happily shredding pieces of bedding, which it will then add to the nest.

Leaving the nest

The next great adventure in the life of a young jird is that first peek out of the nest box, followed by the first few tentative footsteps into the outside world. To us, this is only the inside of a tank or cage but, to the youngster, it is a whole new world. The slightest sound or movement from outside its environment will send it scurrying back to the safety of its nest box.

As a young jird gains confidence, the amount of time spent away from the nest box increases. This is the beginning of independence and also about the time the mother loses interest – her job is almost done.

Young jirds soon emulate their parents. It really is a case of 'Anything you can do, I can do – I think!', as sometimes things do not work out as well as they have planned.

Digging

The next major step during their progression to adulthood is learning to dig. People often think that the animal is trying to dig its way out of the cage but this is not the case. A jird spends a large proportion of its time digging and scratching. This is a natural instinct because in the wild this energy would be put into excavating a burrow – vital in the natural habitat.

Communication

Jirds have an exceptionally effective method of communicating over reasonable distances. This is achieved with the hindlegs. There is no fixed rhythm – it can range from a slow tap, tap, tap to what can only be described as a very fast drum roll. Although there has been no scientific study into this means of communicating, it is believed the changes in tempo represent different messages such as a warning of impending danger, a call to attract a mate, a warning to another jird entering its territory and even just a general greeting.

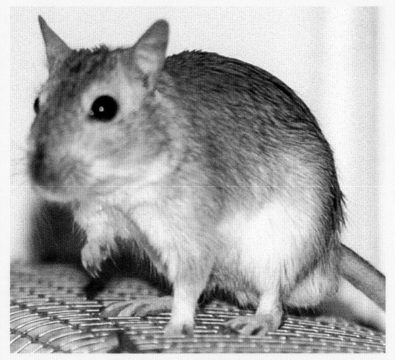

An alert jird on top of its cage.

Marking

One pattern of jird behaviour that you may consider antisocial is the way jirds scent-mark everything with urine and faeces. Males tend to do this more than females. Although sometimes unpleasant, this is a natural part of their behaviour.

Males scent mark anything and everything: cages/tanks, nest boxes, woodshavings, their bedding, and even your hand when you hold them, especially if you have just handled another jird. Females scent very little in comparison.

Grooming

Jirds are very clean animals and I have never come across one that will foul its own nest.

A healthy jird will always be well groomed. It uses its front paws and tongue to wash its face, ears, head, tail and body. This not only promotes cleanliness but also stimulates the skin, prevents the fur from becoming matted and keeps the coat shiny and looking healthy.

Grooming the fur stimulates the skin to produce the natural oils that prevent it from becoming dry and flaky. All jirds have a slightly oily texture to their fur, which helps to repel water. If a jird's fur becomes wet, it will roll about and rub itself on any suitable material it can find in an effort to dry its fur.

You will often see jirds grooming each other. I feel that this is a means of bonding, of showing a partner or another jird that it has been accepted.

Agility

Jirds have extremely powerful hindlegs and are adept at jumping, running and climbing. I have often observed my jirds jump from a sitting position to heights of 37.5–45cm (15–18in). This is an extraordinary feat when you consider that the animal has an average body length of 14cm (5.5in). Starting from running, a jird can achieve even greater heights.

It is essential that your jird spends some time out of its cage, a time it will use to its best advantage. No rodent confined to a cage can exercise fully and jirds are particularly active creatures.

Most jirds are dare-devils. They will attempt to climb almost any surface. They have extremely long nails, enabling them to grip and climb seemingly impossible objects. I once watched one of my jirds scale a vertical louvre door with ease. They have no apparent fear of heights.

A first-time jird owner will probably panic when his or her pet decides to show off its acrobatic skills. Usually your jird will be fine, and you should only intervene when it is in danger of falling or hurting itself. More often than not, a jird will amaze you with its ability to get itself out trouble.

Needless to say, jirds do sometimes get themselves into dangerous situations through no fault of their own. I would advise any pet owner to be vigilant at all times.

General posture

Usually jirds run around on all four feet, using their short front legs for balance and support. They sometimes stand upright on their hind legs much like prairie dogs. To eat they squat in a semi-upright position. Their tails help them balance whilst they are standing, sitting and jumping.

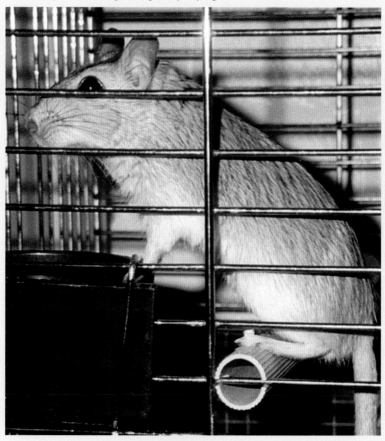

Using front feet for support.

HEALTH

Jirds are healthy and robust rodents. If the owner adheres to a strict cleaning and feeding regime, a jird should live a long, healthy, happy, active life. The average lifespan is two to three years, but exceptionally a jird can reach five.

Most veterinary practices do not specialise in small animals, so it is worth while telephoning different veterinary surgeons to find out who is the most suitable for your pet's needs. When you find a suitable vet, ask him or her to give your pet a full check-up. This should include the ears, the incisors (as these grow continuously throughout the animal's life and should not be allowed to become overgrown) and looking for any lumps or bumps. Ask your vet's advice about any concerns you have for your pet.

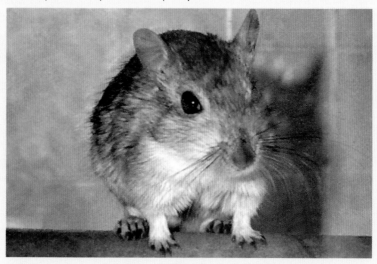

The picture of health: a five-week-old jird.

Occasionally, a jird can suffer from respiratory problems or sore eyes, but more often than not this is caused by the use of fine sawdust as floor covering. Changing to woodshavings normally resolves the problem in a very short time.

Sometimes a jird can suffer from ear problems, usually because it has caught the fleshy part of the ear with its claws while scratching and the wound has become infected. This will require treatment by a vet.

Probably the most serious condition likely to affect a jird is a scent gland tumour. This can be treated successfully if caught in the early stages. Jirds usually come through the anaesthetic quite well.

Keeping health records

It is as essential to keep health records as it is to keep breeding records. Have a card for each jird and list any illness it has suffered throughout its life. An accurate medical history can often help your vet to diagnose the problem.

YOUR FIRST SERIES

The *Your First* series aims to introduce new and would-be owners to the species of their choice. Despite its modest price, each book contains all the information the first-time buyer needs to embark on his or her new hobby and is lavishly illustrated with colour photographs.

Aquarium	185279 052 0	YFK100
Budgerigar	185279 051 2	YFK102
Canary	185279 037 7	YFK103
Chinchilla	185279 140 3	YFK511
Chipmunk	185279 121 7	YFK508
Cockatiel	185279 038 5	YFK104
Dwarf Hamster	185279 122 5	YFK509
Fancy Rat	185279 056 3	YFK501
Ferret	185279 046 6	YFK105
Finch	185279 049 0	YFK106
Gerbil	185279 039 3	YFK107
Giant African Land Snail	185279 057 1	YFK502
Goldfish	185279 040 7	YFK108
Guinea Pig	185279 041 5	YFK109
Hamster	185279 042 3	YFK110
Kitten	185279 055 5	YFK118
Koi	185279 059 8	YFK504
Lizard	185279 043 1	YFK111
Lovebird	185279 045 8	YFK112
Millipede and Cockroach	185279 082 2	YFK505
Mouse	185279 048 2	YFK120
Parrot	185279 044 X	YFK113
Pond	185279 081 4	YFK506
Praying Mantis	185279 141 1	YFK512
Puppy	185279 054 7	YFK119
Rabbit	185279 050 4	YFK114
Snake	185279 047 4	YFK115
Stick Insect	185279 079 2	YFK507
Terrapin	185279 058 X	YFK503
Tropical Fish	185279 053 9	YFK116

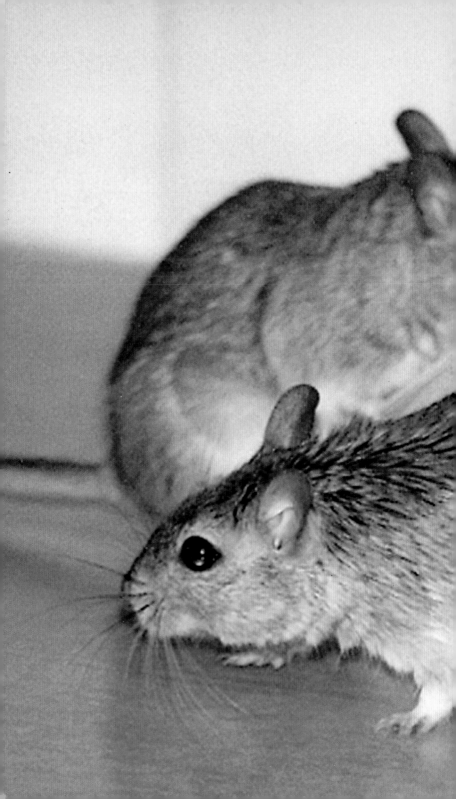